The Magic of Tea

Getting to Know More about the Cup That Cheers

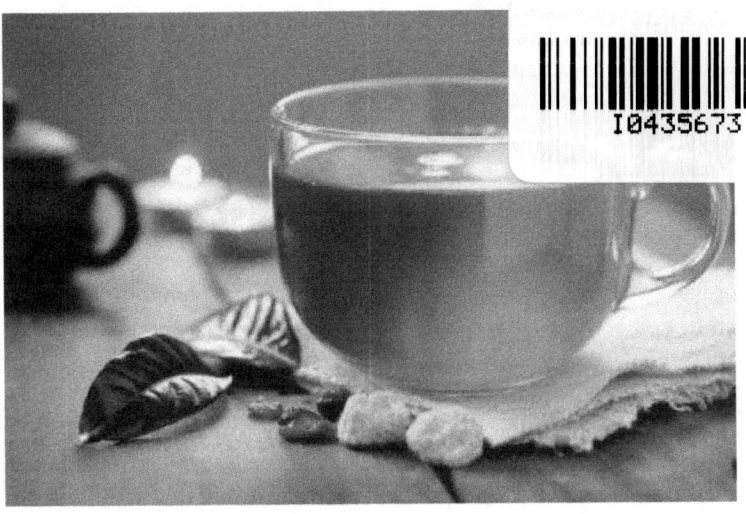

Health Learning Series

Dueep Jyot Singh

Mendon Cottage Books

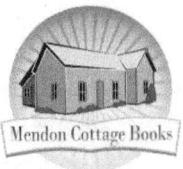

JD-Biz Publishing

Disclaimer

The information is this book is provided for informational purposes only. It is not intended to be used and medical advice or a substitute for proper medical treatment by a qualified health care provider. The information is believed to be accurate as presented based on research by the author.

The contents have not been evaluated by the U.S. Food and Drug Administration or any other Government or Health Organization and the contents in this book are not to be used to treat cure or prevent disease.

The author or publisher is not responsible for the use or safety of any diet, procedure or treatment mentioned in this book. The author or publisher is not responsible for errors or omissions that may exist.

Warning

The Book is for informational purposes only and before taking on any diet, treatment or medical procedure, it is recommended to consult with your primary health care provider.

Our books are available at
1. Amazon.com
2. Barnes and Noble
3. Itunes
4. Kobo
5. Smashwords
6. Google Play Books

Table of Contents

Introduction 4

Growing Tea 11
    Tea cuttings 13

Two Leaves and a Bud.. 15
    Flushes, Banjis and Janams.................................. 15

Harvesting – Plucking, Tipping and Pruning.............. 18

Processing Tea 21

Green and Black Tea Processing................................ 22

Fermentation 24

Enemies of Tea... 25

The Art of Drinking Tea 26
    Masala Chai... 27

    Iced tea 27

    Masala lemon tea –... 30

Tea Bags... 32
    Tea bricks.. 33

Storing tea 34

Conclusion 35

Author Bio.. 36

Publisher... 46

Introduction

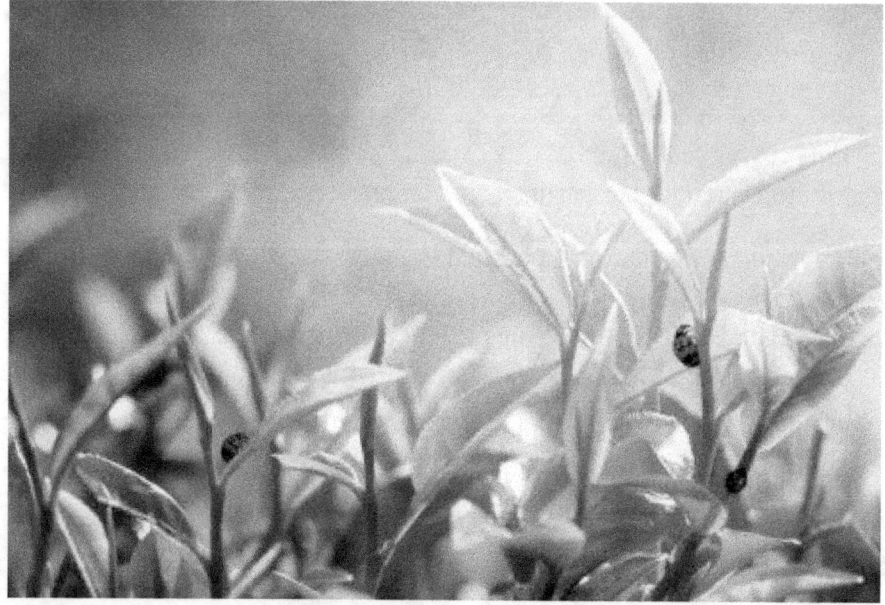

Many of us cannot do without the cup that cheers, first thing in the morning, to wake us up. And whenever we smell the delicious aroma of freshly brewed tea, we thank the person who found out this plant and the brew made from it, which would wake us up and rejuvenate our systems. Why not, this is the refreshing beverage which is consumed gratefully all over the world, second only to water.

According to historical documents, Tea leaves of an evergreen shrub – Camellia sinensis-were steeped in water to make an aromatic beverage in China, more than 4000 years ago. That is because this shrub was first found growing native in Asia.

Even today you can find while the plants growing in many parts of northeastern India, Southwest China, northern Burma, and North Indochina.

This native Chinese tea was slightly bitter, had a cooling effect, and had and astringent and warming flavor. Other tea varieties had floral, sweet, grassy, and even nutty overtones and flavors.

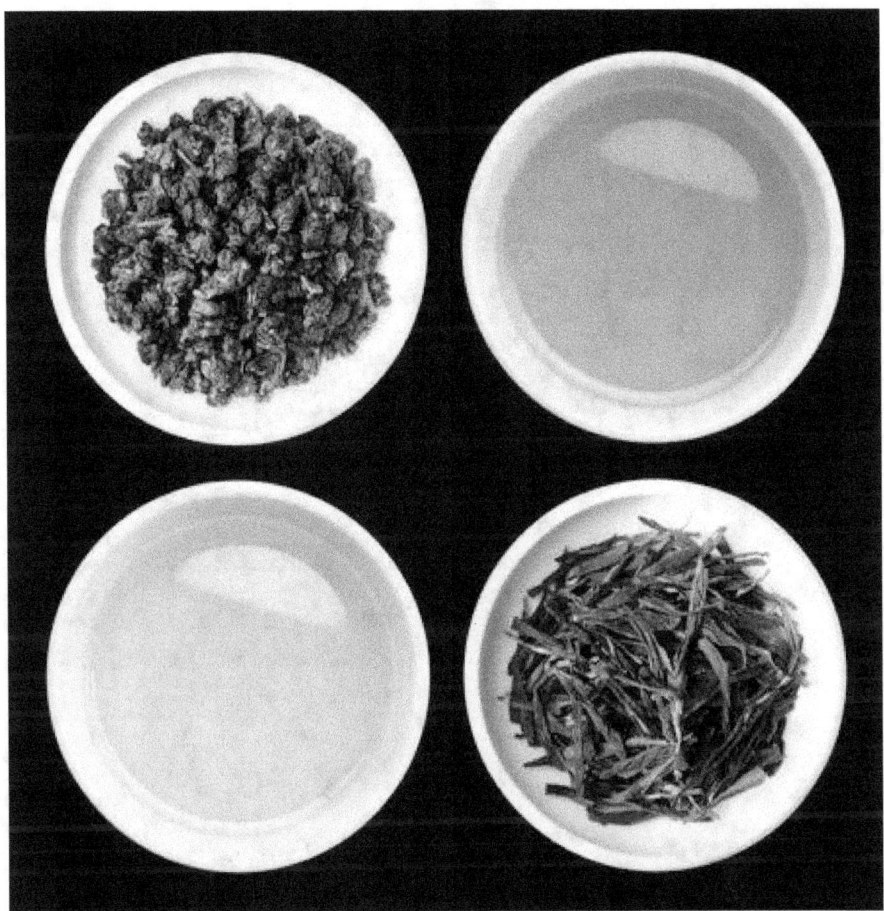

Some historians say that tea has been comparatively lucky when compared to the native ginkgo plant. Tea was cultivated and that is why it managed to survive. Ginkgo stayed wild and that is why it is now in the rare and vanishing species category.

The ancient Chinese drank tea as a medicinal restorative drink. It was only about 3000 years ago, that they began brewing tea as a stimulating drink, without the addition of herbs and leaves and began to drink it as a brew. At this time, it was called t'i [bitter herb] or ch'a depending on the area in which it was grown. It appeared in the West, in the 16th century, through Portuguese merchants and up to the 17th century it was considered to be an exotic drink available only to the rich who could afford it.

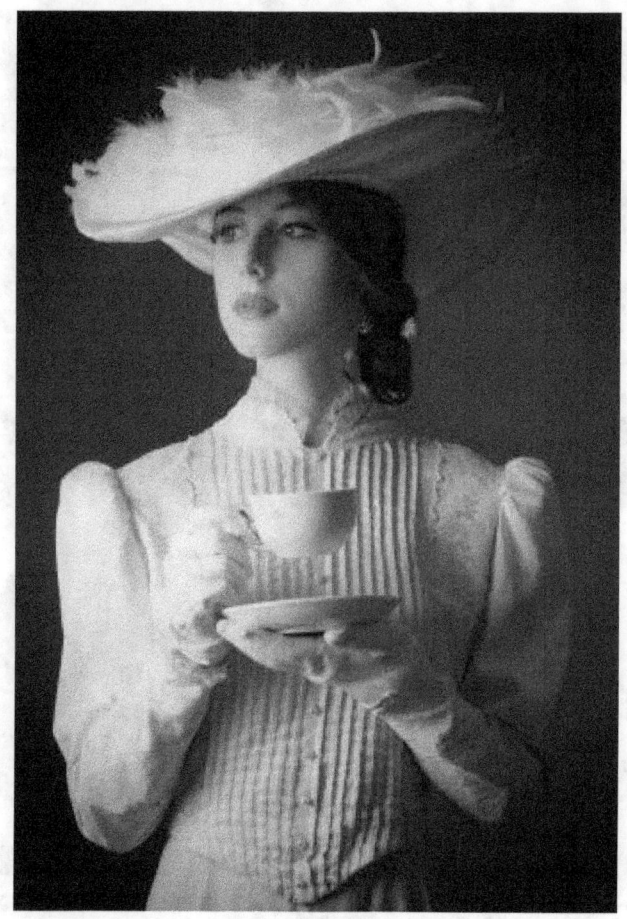

Tea plantations were introduced on the Indian subcontinent by the British rulers in the 17th and 18th century. It began to be grown extensively in Darjeeling and in Sri Lanka, the then Ceylon. This was their way of trying to break the Chinese monopoly on the exportation of tea. Exporting this tea from India in large quantities made it accessible to the general public, and that is why, tea as a luxury item became tea, the drink of the masses.

Apart from tea leaves, herbal teas have also been well known as restorative warming beverages. These teas are normally called tisanes and have been in existence for millenniums. These teas are herbal infusions made up of herbs, fruit, roots, leaves, seeds, and other parts of the plants steeped in hot water and fed to patients. These are completely herb-based and do not have anything to do with the beverage which we know as tea.

It is surprising to know that even though the British made India one of the largest exporters of tea in the 18th and 19th century all over the world, the common folk did not know much about this brew. My father who was born in a remote village, recalls that it was in the early 40s that Britishers decided to market tea in India with a campaign of a colored advertisement of a man sniffing the aroma of fragrant tea and saying "what a beautiful aroma!" Until then, milk and hard drinks were the only brew which was drunk by the people of that area and tea was the preferred brew of Anglicized Indians. And thus the natives living in villages and small towns of India were introduced to tea in the 20th century!

Coffee, of course, was unknown to those people. We have to thank the extensive tea popularizing campaign launched by the Indian tea board to get people to know about this drink, during this time.

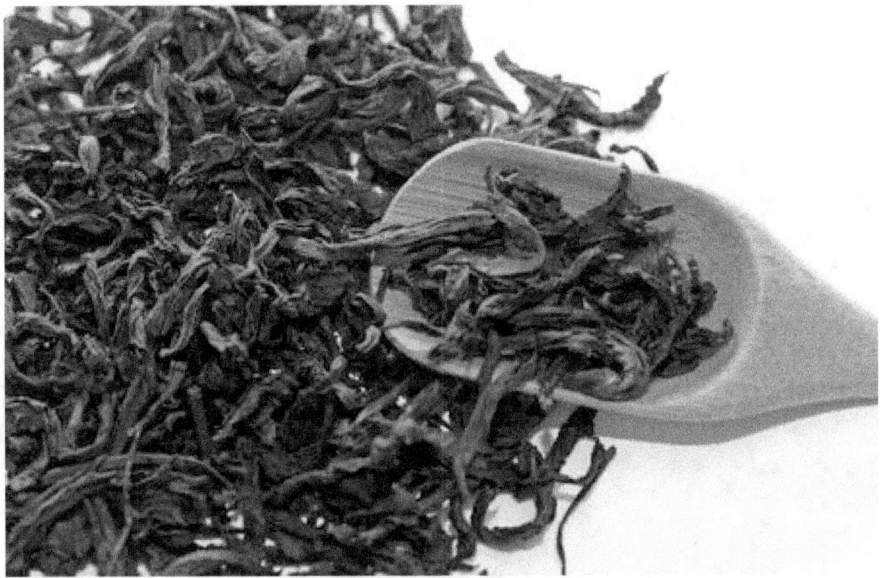

And so tea began to be drunk as a warming beverage in the Indian subcontinent by the common people, even though ancient historical and medical treatises talk about tea as a medical infusion being used down the centuries by people in that land, as well as other parts of the East.

I still remember my grandmother telling us kids, "Tea is not a drink to be given to young children. It is for grown-ups." And "if you drink tea as a child, you are going to grow dark and dusky in complexion!"

As a fair complexion was considered to be very desirable – as it still is, in many parts of the world today, – we children kept away from tea. It was not a drink for children, unless one wanted to look as dark as the tea! In fact, I took that bit of preventative threat to a higher level and do not drink any stimulating beverage, including tea or coffee, even now. [By choice. I cannot see why people like to drink a bitter boiling hot brew every four hours.] But that did not stop me from getting irritated when my colleagues at work wanted regular tea and coffee breaks, because they could not work without those artificial stimulants.

So remember a non-tea drinker is a misfit in any sort of social gathering. That is because tea has become such an integral part of our social lives that we cannot do without it.

Tea is known all over the world today as tea, cha or chai – the yi suffixed being added to cha somewhere in the 17th century, when tea was introduced in the Persian, Turkish, and Arabian, and Central Asian market. So where is my cup of hot chai?

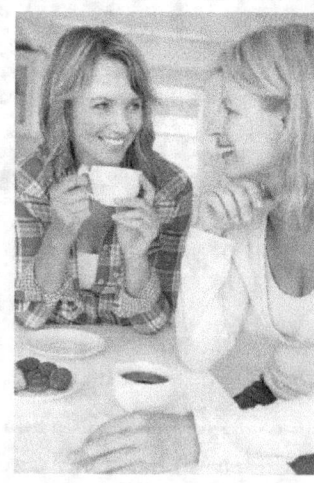

According to Chinese legend, a priest named Shennong used this brew in order to keep awake around 4700 years ago. Medical treatises dating back to 1700 years ago speak about the power of the "bitter t'u , which helps one to think better." That was the tannin in the tea working overtime.

Just like coffee, tea also happens to be a stimulating drink which prevents people from sleeping. That is why it began to be drunk extensively in China by brain workers, who needed to work on treatises long through the night with a clear brain.

In India the power of the tea to keep you awake was mostly appreciated by truck drivers who did most of their long haul truck driving during the night. That is why they demanded 300 mile teas and 400 mile teas from the food and drink shops along the road. This powerful concentrated tea prevented them from sleeping on the road.

Even today, if I want to go on a long drive for about eight hours continuously, I am going to ask for a 400 mile tea from the nearest Dhaba who will supply me with a powerful concentrated brew with lots of sugar, and huge amounts of creamy milk. This will keep me awake for the next 10 hours.

It was in 1848 that tea plants was smuggled out of China by an enterprising Britisher to be planted in the Himalayas. The seeds were introduced by them in Northeast India, where they did not grow at all. However, there was another native tea plant, grown extensively in Assam, which was being used by the natives as a medicinal brew. So with these Chinese tea plants and the Assam variety, the growing of tea in India got underway. That was when the East India company asked people from Britain willing to come to India and managed tea plantations. They would be given land free here, on which they could grow tea. They did the same thing in Ceylon.

And so Darjeeling tea, Ceylon tea and Nilgiris tea, began to break the Chinese monopoly of tea to the West.

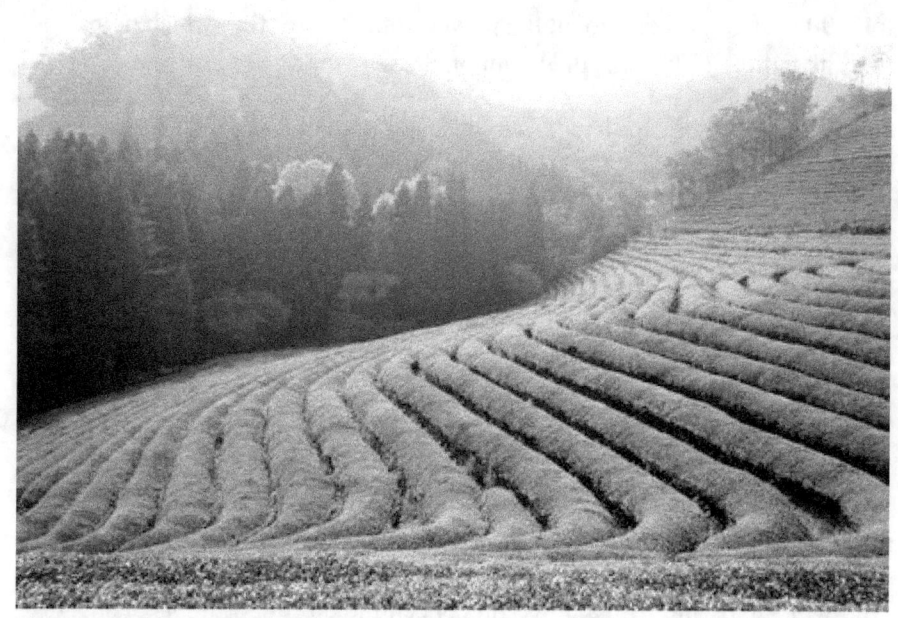

Growing Tea

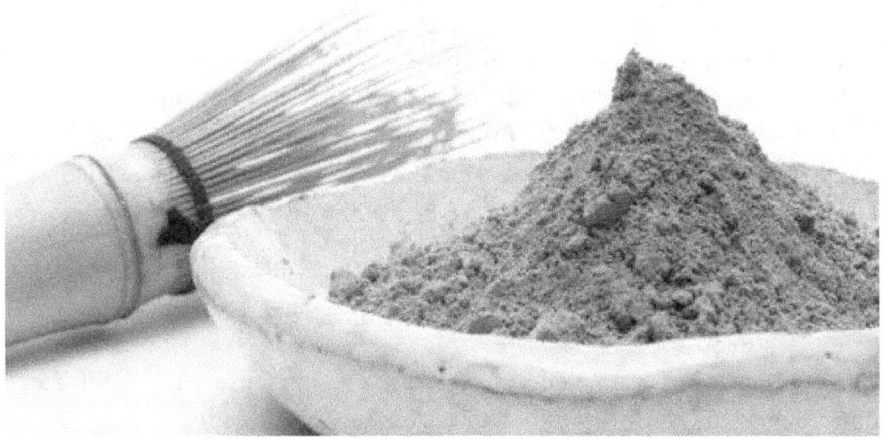

Green tea in powdered form

Tea is rarely propagated vegetatively, except to grow trees to supply seed. These seedling strains and varieties are called jats in India and Ceylon. Sometimes tree to supply seeds are propagated by cuttings or drafting from the best yielding bushes in a plantation.

Cuttings, which are about 12 years old can begin to bear seed for the propagation of more tea plants. It takes three years for a plant to reach maturity enough for harvesting.

The tea plants grown in Assam can become trees instead of remaining as shrubs that is, if you do not prune them. These trees can grow up to 50 feet in height and the leaves can be as much as 12 inches long with 12 – 15 pairs of veins. You may also find the distance between the leaves on shoots of trees which have been pruned for plucking to be as much as 6 inches.

On the other hand, shrubs of the variety bohea do not become nearly so tall and the leaves are only about 2 inches long. These dimensions are of course going to be different in different environments and different jats.

Any tea tree which is growing in a favor and situation and uninjured by diseases, insects, or severe plucking and pruning is going to be long-lived, living up to 60 years

Tea trees prefer growing in a climate, where there is about 50 inches of rainfall per year. The soil needs to be acidic. So a zone 8 climate, or even warmer climate is going to be excellent for growing tea.

The Himalayas were considered to be excellent places in which to grow tea, because they like growing in high places, especially on elevations up to 1500 m above sea level. That means about 5000 feet above sea level. Though the plant growth is slower, the flavor of the tea is enhanced and much more subtle.

The major tea plant varieties grown in China, Formosa, Ceylon and India are Camellia sinensis, Camellia s. var assamica, etc.

The seeds may be germinated in sand and planted in nursery beds until the outer shells crack. The hard shell of the tea seed impedes the water penetration and germination somewhat by giving protection to the embryo.

You can also plant the seeds directly in beds of Sandy soil well worked to a depth of a foot or more, in the shade and watered carefully.

Traditionally nursery seedlings may be planted when they are about six months old. The largest is cut back to stumps, 4 –6 tall. Other seedlings should have all the leaves and part of the stem that still has green color cut off to reduce wilting.

In Formosa, very young plants have the growing tips pinched out to force low branching.

The holes should be 18 – 20 inches deep, and they should be made some months before and left to weather. The filling around the young trees in these holes should be with good and well fertilized topsoil.

Sometimes you may see roots forming on young defoliated trees before new leaves open. Trees are planted three – 5 feet apart in a row, the distances greater for stronger growing jats, but usually close planting of these trees result in higher yields.

Nowadays, some growers are planting hedgerows where the plants are 2 ½ feet apart in a row. This brings the planting to full leaf sooner and is expected to be more convenient for mechanical harvesting.

Tea cuttings

Cuttings before planting, containing one leaf, and a bud do very well in nursery and peat soil, if it is rich in organic matter and has good texture and is below pH 7.

If you are trying to get cuttings from bushes, cut them level across and the new shoots should be permitted to grow until the stems begin to turn red at the bases and become woody. These are now taken and the succulent apical parts and the wooden basal parts are discarded.

The remaining part of the shoot is then made into cuttings, each containing an internode with a bud and a subtending leaf at the apex.

These cuttings have to be planted before they have time to wilt. They will not "take" if they are stored more than a few hours. Tea plants need lots of watering, but the water should not be allowed to stagnate. They tend to be rooted and start shoot growth in about three months .

Shade should then be gradually reduced to harden them for planting in the field. This may be about nine months after the cuttings have been made after routing these cuttings seem to grow about as fast as seedlings and they can also survive dry weather, as well as plantings.

Tea plants are mainly classified by the size of their leaves. The largest tea leaves belong to the variety grown in Assam, the smallest leaves are the ones grown in China and intermediate sized leaves grow in Formosa and Cambodia.

Tea plants are basically trees, and can grow to more than 52 feet, as in Assam where they grow wild. However, they are pruned very often, so that they remain shrubs. This makes it easier for a person to pluck the tea leaves. These shrubs come up to the height of one's waist or a little above.

Also plants that are shorter are going to bear more leaves and thus yield more tea of high quality.

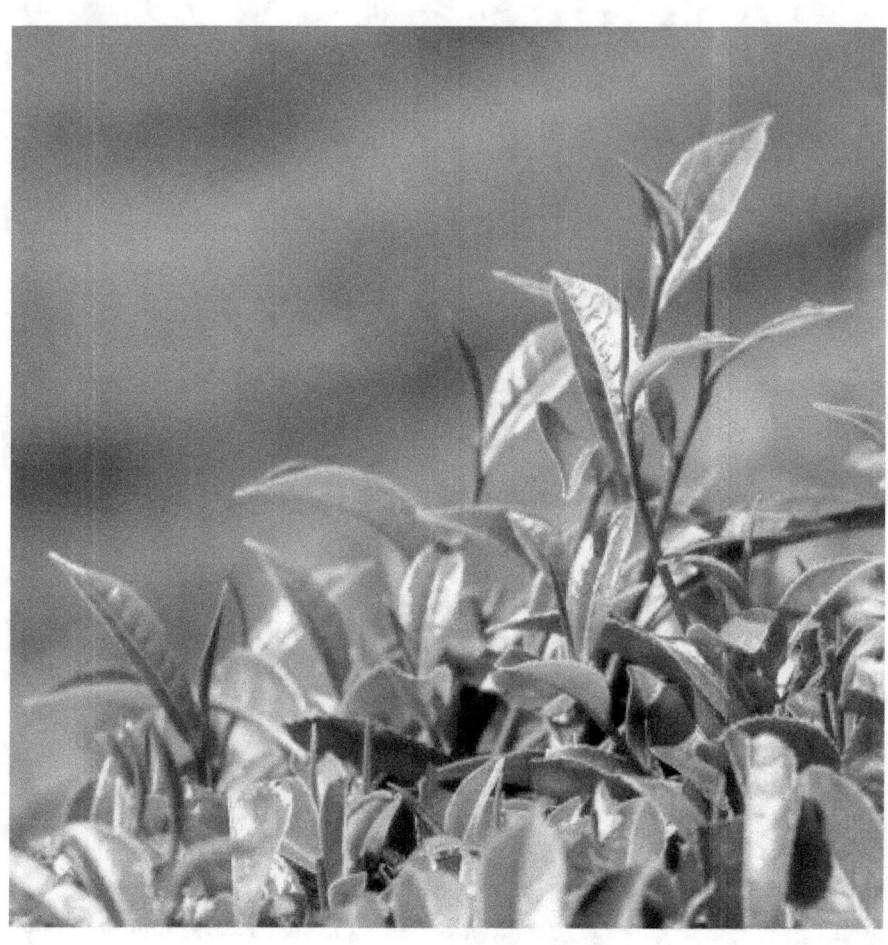

Two Leaves and a Bud

The tea which we loved to drink is the succulent shoot tip with the young expanding leaves. The youngest part of this contains hair that become yellow under the treatments that turn older leaves black. These yellow hair in the black leaf mass are known as the tips. Any tea sample with many tips is valued highly.

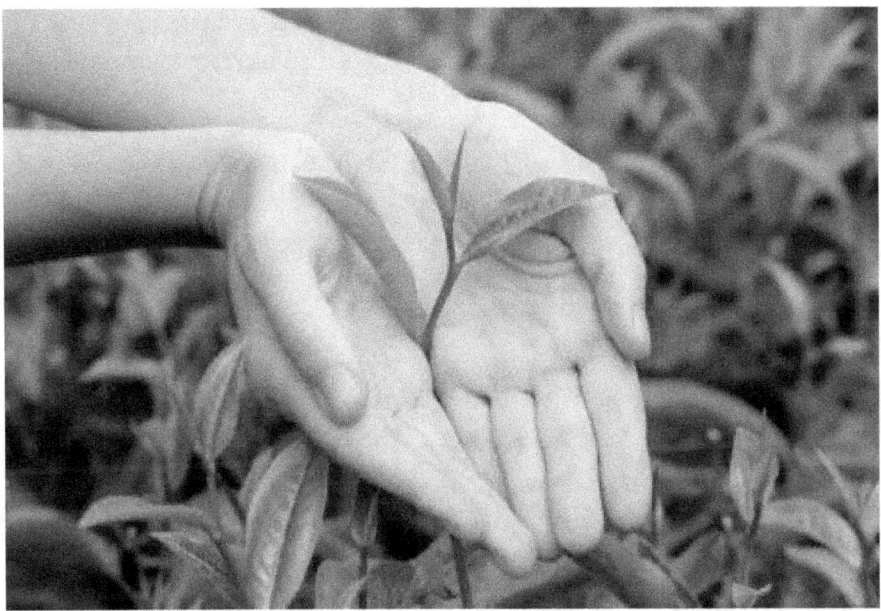

Flushes, Banjis and Janams

These tips grow on the top 2 inches and are plucked with the thumb and forefinger. A growing shoot with an expanding bud and expanding young leaves is called a flush.

Flushes grow every two weeks during spring and the other favorable growing seasons. Traditionally, in India and Ceylon, this picking is still being done by hand, even though in Japan and Russia, shears are being used.

In Ceylon, the plucking is done below the second expanded leaf from a growing bud. The quality of tea is reduced when older leaves are included in this picking. The shoot is plucked back to the bud at the uppermost leaf left. The piece of stem between this leaf and the lowest one taken is then discarded.

A bud that fails to grow is called a Banji. Traditionally, one normal leaf is left on a shoot at plucking. Below this normal leaf is one leaf much smaller than normal. This is known as the fish leaf or janam the first leaf out of the but is still smaller than the fish leaf and it is going to fall soon.

A stronger flash can grow from a bud at a normal leaf, but the flush is going to grow from the Bud at the fish leaf or even from the bud, at the smaller first leaf – the one that falls – if the shoot is pinched back to that particular bud.

When the shoot is plucked back to the bud at the fish leaf, this plucking must be done while the shoot is younger, and when it has only two instead of three expanded leaves. This means plucking needs to be more frequent.

This plucking is known as hard plucking.

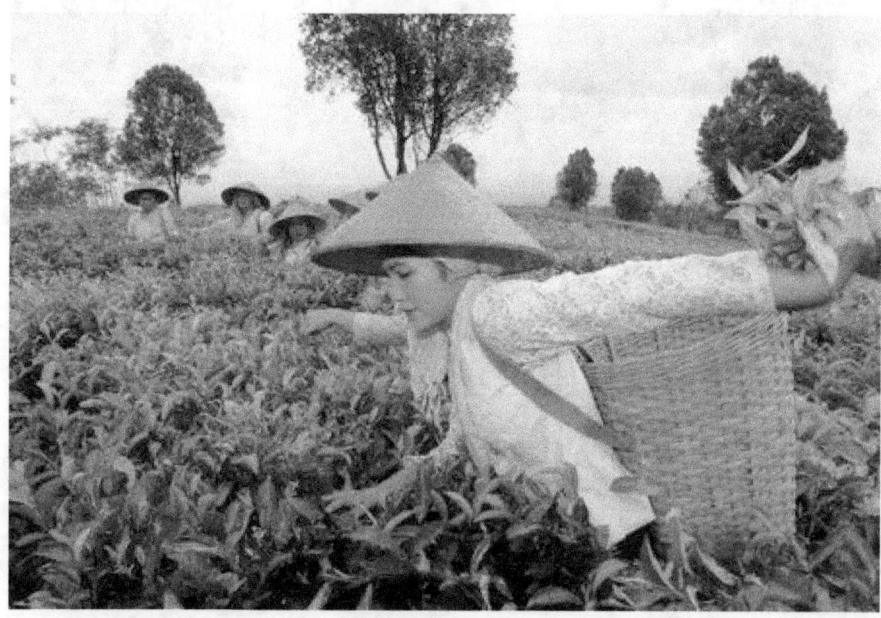

After this plucking is done, the only leaf surfaces left on the tree are those on the shoots before the plucking table along the branches. The shoots may not always be at the right stage for plucking at one time and so the pluckers inspect all the plants regularly in order to get all the flushes that are approximately at the right condition.

The frequency of this plucking is going to depend on the rate of flush growth, about every week for trees on good soil in warm climates like Ceylon. It can also be every two weeks or later, when the mean daily temperature is considerably lower as in places at higher elevations.

For places where tea is grown near the equator, plucking is done throughout the year, with a lower yielding in the cool and dry months.

Harvesting – Plucking, Tipping and Pruning

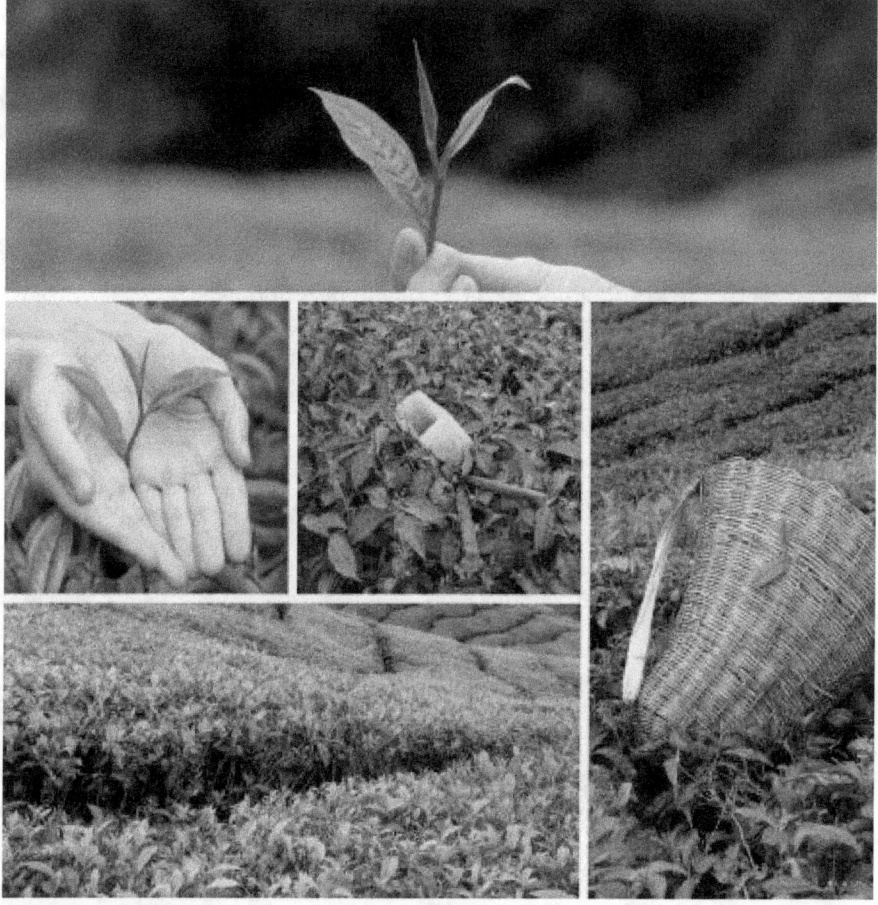

For careful plucking the top of the hedge row of the trees should be nearly level. You should also have a flat plucking table, which is at a convenient height for the pluckers. This cannot be done by amateurs, because this needs careful training. Plucking alone will not keep enough buds flushing and increased numbers of bud become banji. That is why to renew the flushing of the trees, as well as to keep the plucking table down to a suitable height, severe pruning is done regularly.

You can consider plucking also to be a rather severe form of pruning. All this pruning naturally has a pronounced influence on the psychology of the plant in other ways than merely dwarfing it. This may also influence the quality of the product.

After pruning the new shoots should not be plucked when they have 3 leaves above the fish leaf. However, you can pinch them or break them back to a certain distance from the ground – 18 – 24 inches – or 6 – 9 inches above the central pruning cut. This process is called tipping instead of plucking.

You may need to do several tippings before you can get a good plucking table.

Delaying the first tipping until a considerable leaf surface has been formed is going to cause the first flush after the pruning to show a less reduction in quality than if the plucking has been done earlier, while the shoots were more succulent.

In this tipping two or more normal leaves are left above the fish leaf, whenever this stub does not project above the height at which the plucking table is being formed.

The greater number of leaves left with their buds is to obtain more branches to form a plucking table.

The time between the pruning and the first tipping is going to depend upon the severity of the pruning, the variety of the jat, the fertility of the soil and how favorable the temperature is for the rapid growth of the shoots. This can be six weeks to four months.

The pluckings are collected in baskets by each worker and must be weighed in for processing, several times during a day whether the basket is full or not. On the plant or in a shallow layer in the basket such shoots are going to have approximately the temperature of the air. But towards the center of a considerably deeper mass in the basket the heat of respiration or of fermentation is not going to escape. This may accumulate to injurious temperature and may cause injury to the shoots through fermentation.

The green weight of plucking by one person in a day is going to depend, not merely on the speed of the worker, but also on the flushing of the jat in the environment concerned. 25 pounds or more in high jats in a favorable situation for growth can also be as low as 5 pounds in low producing jats at higher elevations.

Processing Tea

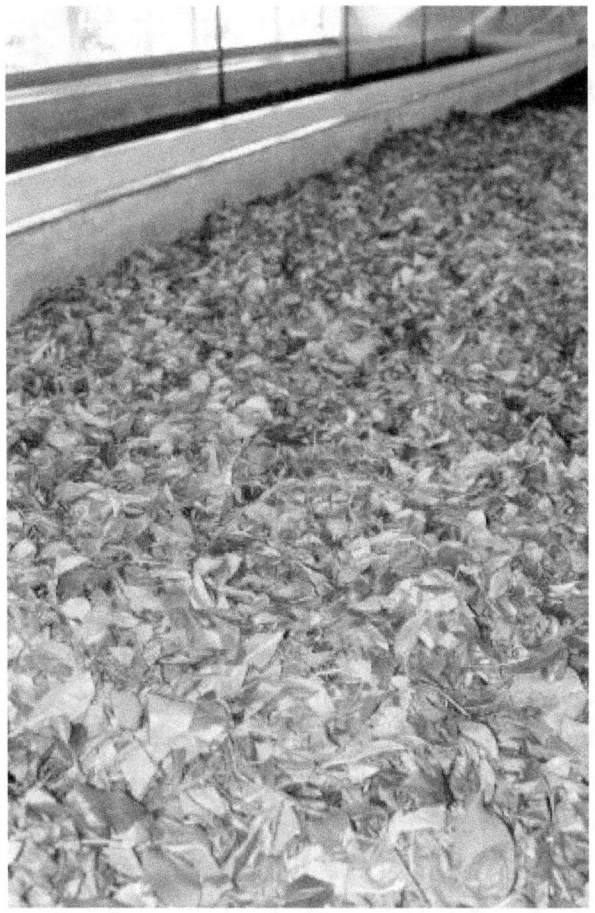

The tea that you commonly get in the market is of six types. The white tea is going to be unoxidized and wilted. Yellow Tea are leaves which have been allowed to turn yellow, even though they are unoxidized and unwilted.

Green tea which is so popular in social tea drinking ceremonies in China and Japan is unoxidized and unwilted.

Oolong tea which is bruised, wilted and oxidized partially is considered to be an expensive and luxury tea. The normal black tea is wilted tea which has been oxidized fully, and sometimes crushed. It is also known as red tea in India and China. This is normally used in traditional medicine.

In China, black tea is that tea which has been allowed to ferment or turn into "compost."

Fermentation /oxidization of the leaves, as well as the time taken to oxidize them is going to create the product which you bring home from the supermarket shelves.

These leaves start to wilt and ferment unless they are dried immediately Many of the processes in getting the ready can be considered to be more engineering than horticulture.

We know that tea is grown mainly for its stimulating tannin content. We also know that it has a little bit of caffeine in it. In the manufacture of black tea, a small quantity of essential oils are formed, and these oils are what gives your tea such a pleasant odor.

The stimulating effect of a tease due to caffeine, but the quality of the tea is going to be based on the flavor and the appearance given largely by the tea tannin compounds.

Tea of high-quality is going to be richer in these compounds than tea of low quality. These are normally found more in the young leaves, which are chosen for plucking when compared to older leaves or those leaves on Banji shoots.

Green and Black Tea Processing

A considerable amount of green tea is produced in China and Japan. This is not necessarily from different varieties than those used for the making of black tea but is made entirely due to different processing methods.

The leaves needed to make green tea are heated as quickly as possible after harvest to a temperature that inactivates the enzyme, which causes oxidization or fermentation. It is then cooled and rolled and by further heating and rolling it dries eventually to about 4% of moisture.

Green tea is more powerful, because it has more catechins. That is why it is going to be a little more bitter than black tea.

During the processing of black tea, the leaves are first wilted in shallow layers in special drying sheds through which air is circulated. In very humid districts air is warmed a little to reduce the humidity content. This process is known as withering. The withering temperature should be around 90°F. If the temperature is above this the leaf is going to turn red and black.

In rapid wilting the leaves lose water much faster than the stem and they may shrivel up and black and much before the stem tissue has withered. In slower withering, – 12 to 24 hours –, the loss of water from the stems and leaves is more nearly equal.

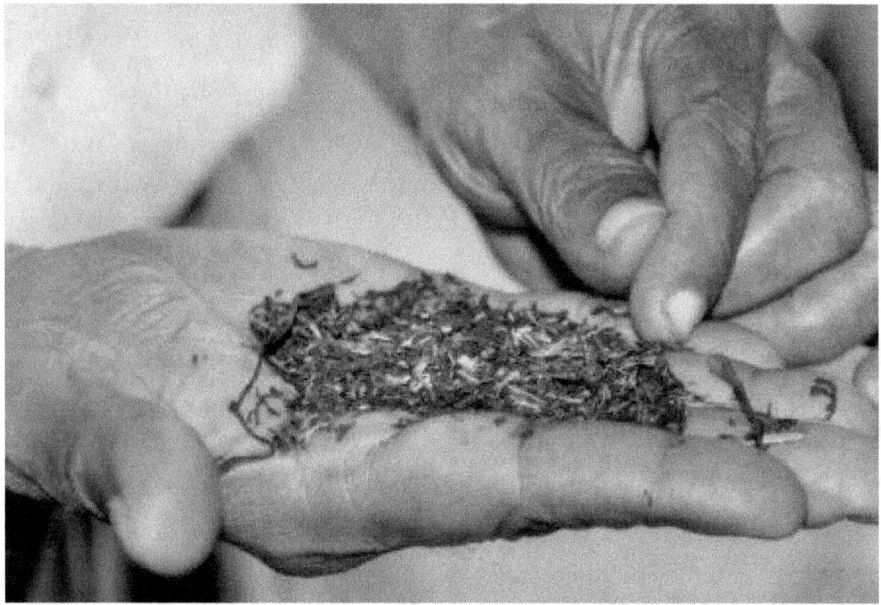

Withering is done so that the leaves when rolled by a twisting or wringing motion to bring the juice to the surface will retain the curled up form given to them. This is the form preferred in the markets. If the pluckings as they come from the fields are still left a little wet, this withering process prevents the bacterial action on the leaves from producing substances that give an unpleasant flavor to the tea.

This tea is then rolled so that some of the juice gets to the surface and comes in contact with the air. A number of rollings are given to the leaves during the processing process.

Fermentation

Fermentation is also known as oxidation. The crushed pluckings are spread loosely over a tile floor about 2 inches thick in height. The temperature is around 86°F during this fermentation process and the first fermentation time is going to be about three hours. After that, the next stage of fermentation is going to be done between 70° to 80°F. If it is more than 90°F. The holiday is going to fall. This fermentation causes the catechin present in the tea to make a thicker liquor when it is added to water. It also sets to develop the aromatic oil, which will be released during the boiling process.

This tea infusion made from fermented tea is pungent, rather than bitter.

Oxidation is going to be stopped at a temperature of 160 – one 90°F depending on the quality of tea you want. In China and Formosa, when oolong tea is being prepared, little bit of fermentation is done before the leaf is heated to inactivate the fermentation, enzyme, but not as much as it is done in the making of black tea. So you can consider oolong tea to be midway between green tea and black tea.

Tea grows best in soil which has a large percentage of nitrogen. That is why in many parts of the East, legumes are also planted near trees, so that the soil stays well supplied with nitrogen. Funnily enough, this was a tradition which people are forgetting especially in research tea plantations in many parts of the world.

Enemies of Tea

There are many fungus diseases as well as viral diseases which can affect a tea harvest. These include blister blight which is caused by a fungus, and infects young leaves. The infected spot is going to show up as a blister on the lower side of the leaf, and a depression on the upper side. This is more prevalent in humid and muggy weather.

Copper blight, Brown blight and gray blight are also caused by fungi. Red rust is caused by algae, which causes red and black spots to show on the upper sides of the leaves and red and gray brown spots showing up on the lower parts.

Using chemical pesticides to control these fungi are definitely not done in the plucking season because that is going to affect the quality of the tea. That is why young trees are sprayed before the plucking table has been formed and the pruned trees are sprayed until flushes for plucking begin to grow.

Insects also cause great losses in tea plantations. Most common of them are hole borers and termites. In Asia, natural pesticides like neem leaf solutions, half a kilo of neem leaves in a gallon full of water is used to spray the leaves, and get rid of all the insects.

The Art of Drinking Tea

Tea, all over the world is considered to be a social stimulant, which can be drunk on ceremonious occasions, or in informal settings. India, Japan and China happen to be the greatest tea drinkers in the world, where drinking tea is a part of social interaction. These ritualized tea ceremonies in Japan and China are normally made with oolong tea

Ordinary tea is made with tea, sugar and milk. In more remote areas of the Indian subcontinent like Ladakh, Tea is mixed with salt and butter and drunk like a soup. In Turkey, tea is going to be served to you in a small glass and is going to be really sweet, like Turkish coffee.

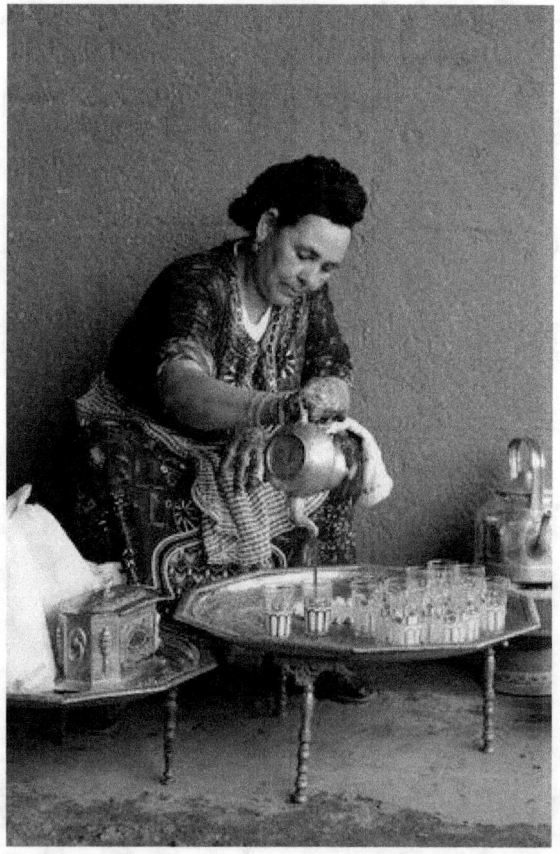

Mint tea in Morocco.

Iced tea and tea bags are a comparatively modern 20th century innovation. You can also get it in decaffeinated form or with tea spices added to it. This is known as masala Chai.

Masala Chai – The spices include cardamom, cinnamon, cloves, pepper and ginger. All of them are put in boiling water, and one tablespoonful of black tea leaves is added to this boiling mixture. It is then left to infuse for 10 minutes. Hot boiling milk is then added, according to taste, and sugar or honey as you wish. This is the popular traditional spicy tea drunk very commonly in many parts of India.

The Irish also love drinking tea, which needs to be hot, sweet and strong. The average consumption of tea drunk every day by the Irish is between 6 to 7 cups. They also like it spicier. Sometimes a little bit of whiskey is also added to the beverage, especially if the drinker has come in from the cold.

Green tea, popularly known as Kahwa is drunk quite commonly with every meal on the silk route of Asia. In Kashmir, the tea may be salty (noon chai) and is going to be made up of cloves, cardamoms, almonds and pistachios. It is also going to be pink in color!

In many parts of Asia, it is a tradition to offer a guest in your house tea with something to eat.

Iced tea – 80% of the tea drunk in the United States is in the form of iced tea. In Switzerland, the Iced-Tea which you are going to drink is going to be made up of mint, lemon juice, sugar and black tea along with native herbs. Peaches and lemon flavors are common. You can also get lemongrass and Jasmine flavors in your choice of iced tea.

In Britain the evening meals are called tea where you are going to be eating cakes, and scones with your brew. This is consumed every day and is important part of British culture. Guests are offered tea, along with cakes and biscuits in the afternoon. If you are visiting the southwest of England, you are going to have scones with clotted cream and jam along with your pot of tea.

You may find this tea arriving to you in a pot covered by a tea cozy. This is to keep the heat in, while the infusion brews in hot water.

I remember an elderly relative who was rather Anglicized. He wanted his tea at 4 o'clock every evening, and that needed fresh cake along with it.

The tea would come to the table in a porcelain pot. It would be covered by a cozy and the tea would be poured by his wife in delicate Wedgewood porcelain cups. After that she would pour just a little bit of milk – boiling hot in a separate white small milk pot – into the tea to change the color from golden brown to creamy brown. One small teaspoon of sugar taken from the sugar container, and his tea was ready to be drunk with warm pieces of cake and scones. He drank his tea with Marie tea biscuits, straight from England, because he did not like the Indian product much! Talk about ritualism!

I naturally, being a kid at that time was given hot creamy milk, with cake, bread, jam/marmalade/Marmite and butter but the ritual in itself was so fascinating that one could understand why the pouring of tea in itself was such a stylish social ceremony.

The traditional method of making tea, in China is to place the leaves directly in the cup. Boiling hot water is then poured directly into the leaves, and this is left to infuse for anywhere between 15 to 20 minutes. In India the tea leaves are added to hot water and allow to boil, infuse and cool before milk and sugar is added directly and another boiling session of one minute is applied. It is then strained and drunk boiling hot.

This brew is going to be strong, depending on the amount of leaves which you are using to make the steeped infusion. Steeping time does not have much effect on the strength of the brew. This steeping time can be anywhere between 9:57 minutes, depending on how you like your tea.

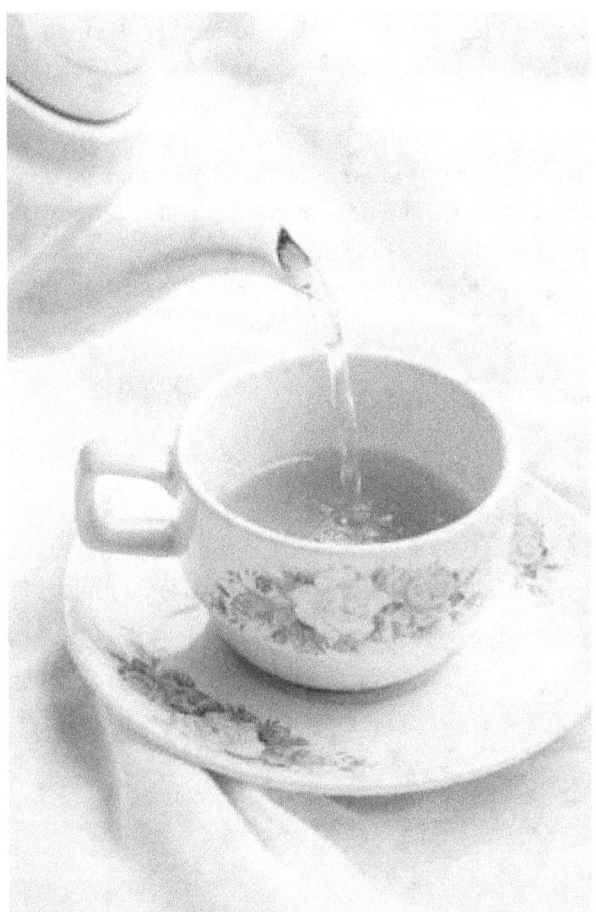

A basic tea recipe is going to be 5 mL – one level teaspoon – for 240 mL or 1 cup of water. You can use lesser quantity of tea leaves to make a delicate Darjeeling tea. However, if you are drinking tea with milk, and you like it strong, you can add more teaspoonfuls of tea to the brew.

Milk was and still is supposed to reduce and neutralize the strength of the tannins in the tea. That is why real tea drinkers do not use milk in their brew.

Brewing temperatures for oxidized teas means boiling – hundred degrees centigrade. Unoxidized teas like oolong, green, yellow and white tea do not need to be boiled. Try simmering them at 65 – 85°C. Green tea temperatures should be around 75 – 80°C and the infusion should be for about two minutes   steeping time. Black tea and flowering tea are boiled and then allow to steep for two minutes.

Oolong tea is one of the teas of which the leaves can be reused. In Chinese ceremonies, the first brew of Oolong is not drunk, because it is considered to be the wash of the leaves. The third brew is considered to be the best of the lot. Steep oolong for about 30 seconds for the first brew, for about one minute for the second brew and for two minutes for the third brew. Then drink this third steeping.

Do not stir the tea when it is infusing.

Masala lemon tea –

This is a new variation of tea, which you can almost considered to be a salty soup. This is going to contain lemon juice, sugar, cinnamon, black salt and roasted cumin seeds. Lemon tea is just ordinary tea with lemon juice and sugar and no milk.

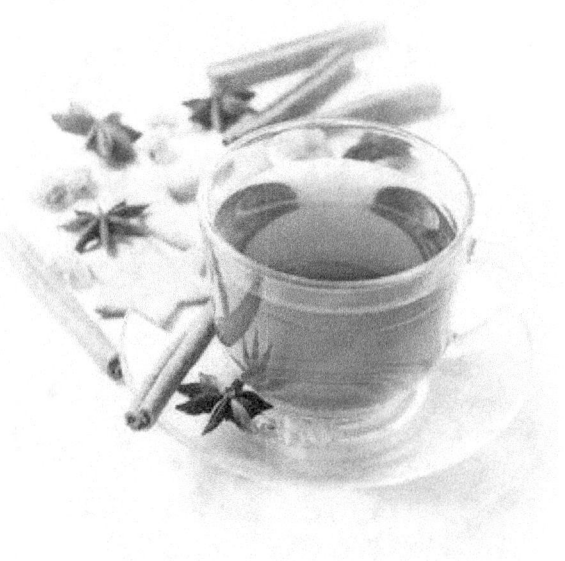

Tea Bags

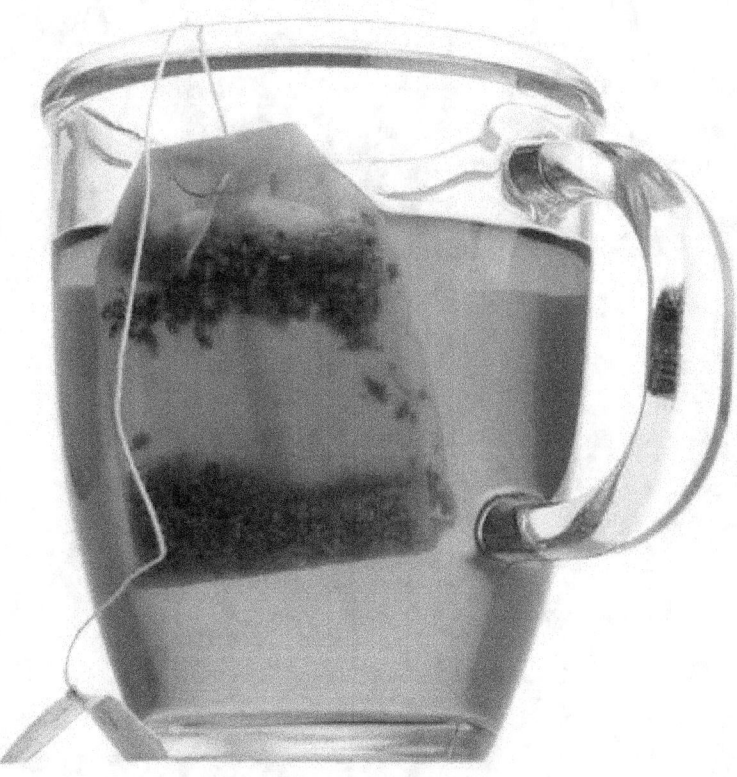

It was in 1907 that an American Thomas Sullivan decided to present his clients with tea samples in small Chinese silk bags. Some of his more enterprising clients found that they could reuse the sample silk bags by replacing the used tea in them. And so they had tea bags ready at hand whenever they wanted to brew a hot cup of Cha. It was only in 1953 that Tetley in UK began to think of making these tea bags and marketing it. They were an immediate hit.

The dust from the leaves were packed into paper bags which allowed them to be steeped in hot water. This gave you a brew of the strength and potency you wish and you did not have to filter the leaves and throw them out either.

The quality of this tea was originally low because it was the dust. However, nowadays, high-quality tea is available in tea bags. Nevertheless, many people do not like teabags because they say that the smaller size of the bag does not allow the tea to percolate and steep in the boiling water. Also, some famous companies' tea bags are not being supported by environmentalists because they considered the bags to be non-biodegradable, when compared to paper bags.

Tea bricks

If you find yourself traveling in Mongolia or in Himalayan countries, you may find your tea in a compressed form. This is called Pu-erh. This compressed tea is excellent for storage, aging and ease of transport. It also stores longer without spoiling.

A bit of this compressed tea is going to be cut off with a knife, brewed in hot water and served to you with butter and salt. So you are going to have tea brick soup. The older this tea is, the more it is going to improving taste and flavor.

Storing tea

Tea needs to be placed in airtight cool, dry and dark places away from any sort of disagreeable odors. You do not want onion flavored tea do you? That is because tea is capable of taking on delicate aromas of ingredients near it are added to it like jasmine flowers and bergamot orange peel.

You can preserve black tea for anywhere between 1 to 2 years if it is placed in a sealed container. Rolled leaves are going to last longer than open leaves. That is why nowadays they are sealed in oxygen absorbing packets by vacuum sealing.

Conclusion

This book introduces you to the magic of tea, the universally acclaimed brew, the cup that cheers. You have got more information on how tea is grown, the types of tea, the way it is processed before it reaches the consumer and the importance of this brew in a social context.

Many people think that the drinking of tea is harmful to health. But then there is always someone who is going to speak his own opinion on any given topic. But since olden times, people know that tea was a medicinal brew which activated the natural detoxification system of the body. It also was supposed to prevent brain cell deterioration and rejuvenated damaged cells.

Black tea was considered to be a blood thinner, preventing blood clots and strokes. White tea like silver Needle and White Peony is comparatively mild in flavor and low in caffeine content. It is supposed to preserve the natural elasticity in your skin and collagen. So if you want to keep youthful, drink white tea, so say the Chinese.

Oolong tea reduces the level of cholesterol and aids in weight loss by boosting up your metabolism. It also reduces clot formation.

So in the words of a famous dancer – Chai is the elixir that feeds my soul. Just like a dancer has to be patient, to internalize the art after learning it, a tea drinker has to wait for the tea to brew well and sip it slowly. The best tea is the one that is never prepared or sipped in a mad rush."

Tea is also considered to be an aid to digestion, while others like it just for the soothing flavor and delicious aroma.

December 15 is international tea Day. So enjoy your cup of tea and your tea break.

Live Long and Prosper!

Author Bio

Dueep Jyot Singh is a Management and IT Professional who managed to gather Postgraduate qualifications in Management and English and Degrees in Science, French and Education while pursuing different enjoyable career options like being an hospital administrator, IT,SEO and HRD Database Manager/ trainer, movie , radio and TV scriptwriter, theatre artiste and public speaker, lecturer in French, Marketing and Advertising, ex-Editor of Hearts On Fire (now known as Solstice) Books Missouri USA, advice columnist and cartoonist, publisher and Aviation School trainer, ex-moderator on Medico.in, banker, student councilor ,travelogue writer … among other things!

One fine morning, she decided that she had enough of killing herself by Degrees and went back to her first love -- writing. It's more enjoyable! She already has 48 published academic and 14 fiction- in- different- genre books under her belt.

When she is not designing websites or making Graphic design illustrations for clients , she is browsing through old bookshops hunting for treasures, of which she has an enviable collection – including R.L. Stevenson, O.Henry, Dornford Yates, Maurice Walsh, De Maupassant, Victor Hugo, Sapper, C.N. Williamson, "Bartimeus" and the crown of her collection- Dickens "The Old Curiosity Shop," and so on… Just call her "Renaissance Woman") - collecting herbal remedies, acting like Universal Helping Hand/Agony Aunt, or escaping to her dear mountains for a bit of exploring, collecting herbs and plants and trekking.

Check out some of the other JD-Biz Publishing books

Gardening Series on Amazon

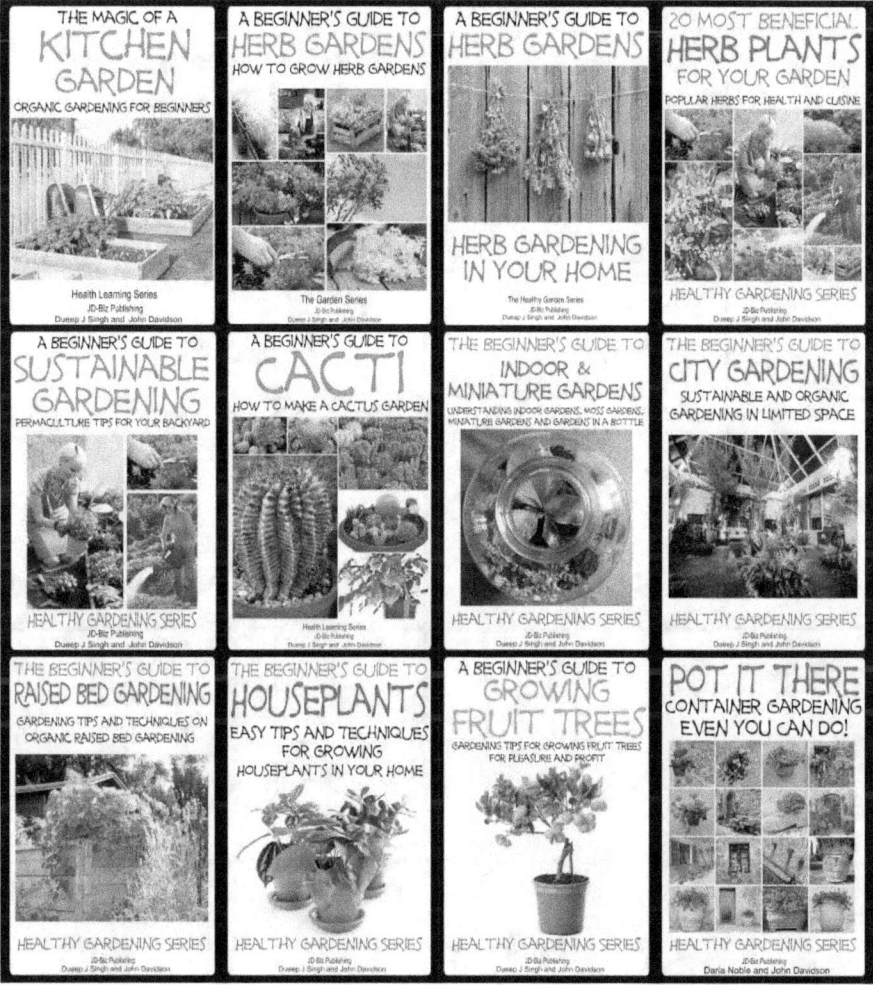

Health Learning Series

THE MAGIC OF GOOSEBERRIES FOR HEALTH AND BEAUTY	THE MAGIC OF YOGURT FOR COOKING AND BEAUTY	THE MAGIC OF LEMONS USING LEMONS FOR HEALTH AND BEAUTY	THE MAGIC OF CHILLIES FOR COOKING AND HEALING	THE MAGIC OF ONIONS ONIONS IN CUISINE TO CURE AND TO HEAL	THE MAGIC OF RADISHES TO CURE AND TO HEAL
THE MAGIC OF CARROTS TO CURE AND TO HEAL	THE HEALTH BENEFITS OF OREGANO FOR COOKING AND HEALTH	THE Magic Of MARIGOLDS Marigolds for Health And Beauty	THE HEALTH BENFITS OF CINNAMON	THE MAGIC OF COCONUTS FOR COOKING & HEALTH	THE MAGIC OF CLOVES FOR HEALINGS AND COOKING
THE MAGIC OF ASAFETIDA FOR COOKINGS AND HEALING	THE MAGIC OF NEEM MARGOSA TO HEAL	THE MAGIC OF SALT TO HEAL AND FOR BEAUTY	THE MAGIC OF POMEGRANATES FOR HEALTH AND BEAUTY	THE MAGIC OF DRY FRUIT AND SPICES REMEDIES AND RECIPES	THE HEALTH BENFITS OF TURMERIC CURCUMIN FOR COOKING AND HEALTH
THE MAGIC OF ALOE VERA	THE MAGIC OF VEGETABLES ANCIENT HEALING REMEDIES AND TIPS	THE HEALTH BENFITS OF ROSEMARY FOR COOKING AND HEALTH	THE MAGIC OF PEPPER & PEPPERCORNS FOR COOKING & HEALING	THE MAGIC OF MILK, BUTTER AND CHEESE FOR COOKING & HEALING	THE MAGIC OF CARDAMOMS FOR COOKING AND HEALTH
THE HEALTH BENFITS OF BLACK CUMIN FOR COOKING AND HEALTH	THE MAGIC OF BASIL-TULSI TO HEAL NATURALLY	THE MAGIC OF SPICES FOR HEALTH AND CUISINE	THE MAGIC OF ROSES FOR COOKING AND BEAUTY	The Miraculous Healing Powers of GINGER	The Miracle of HONEY

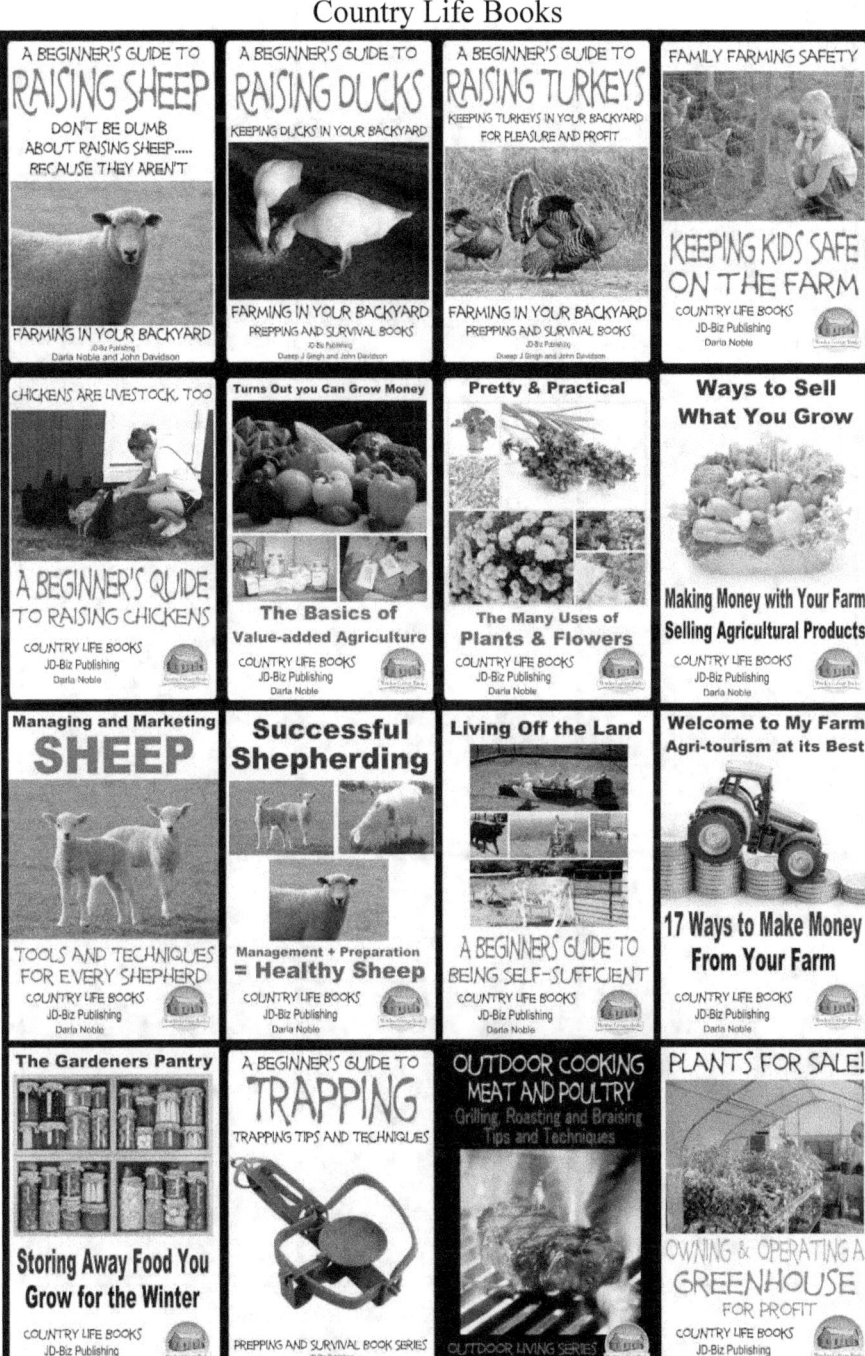

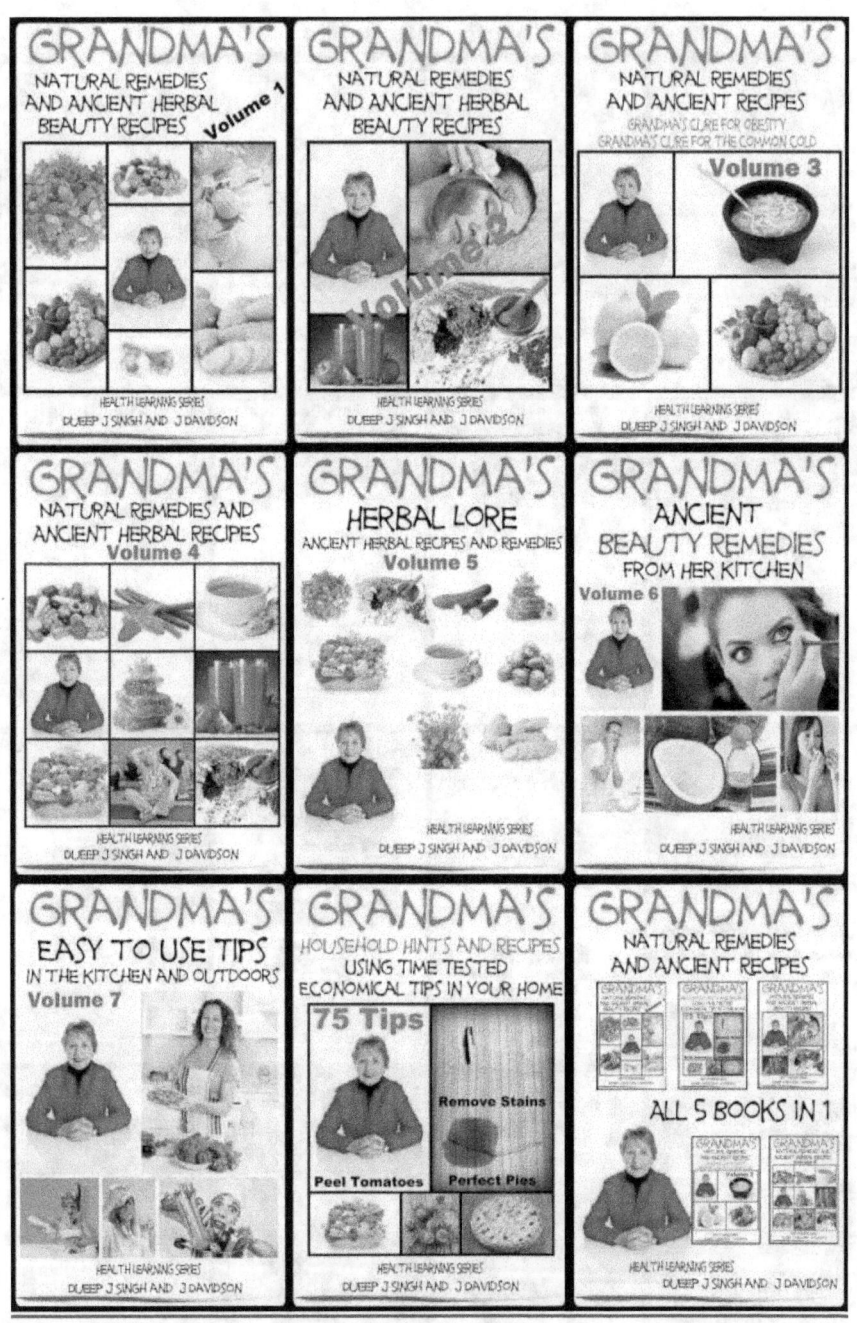

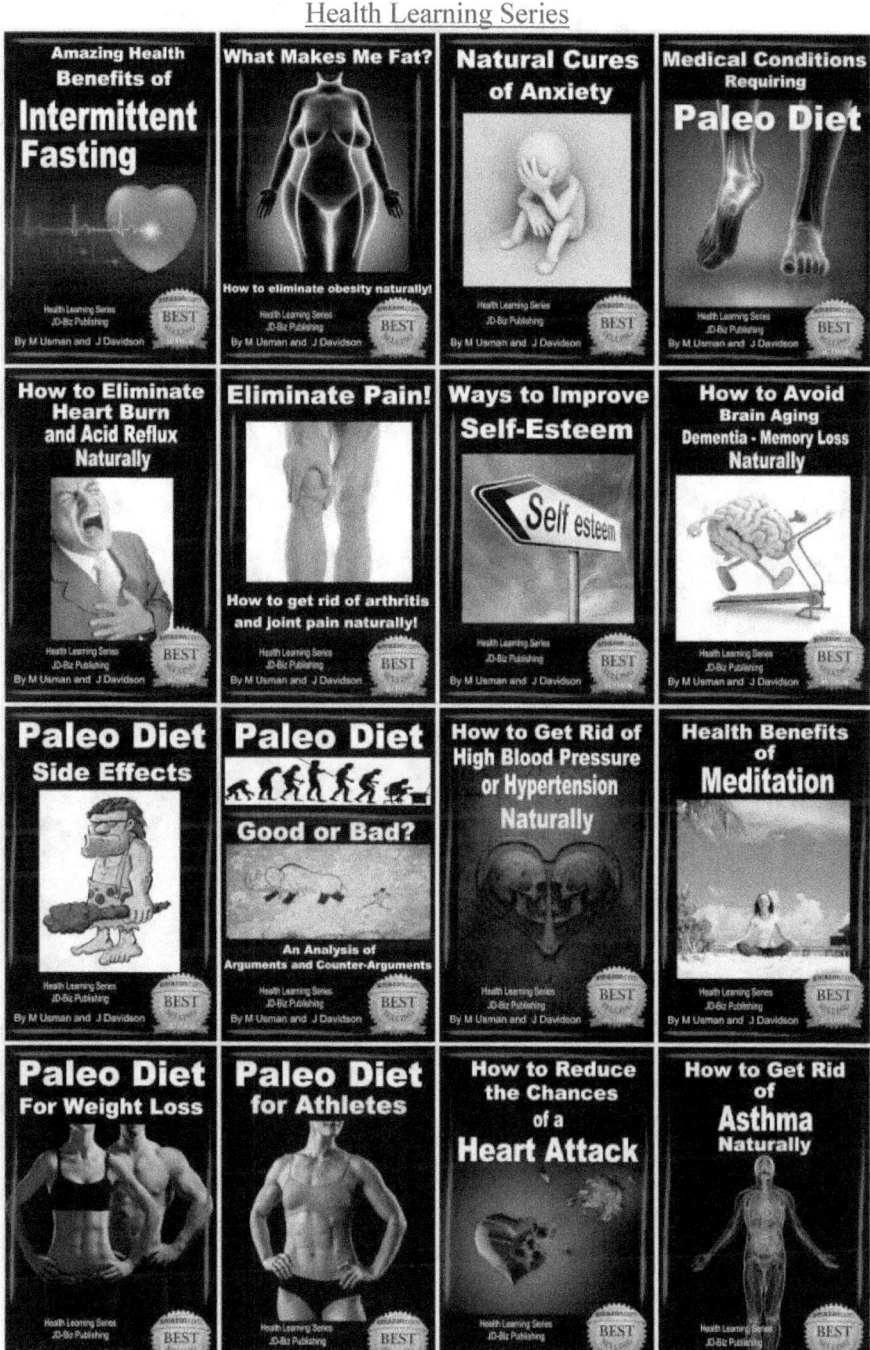

Amazing Animal Book Series

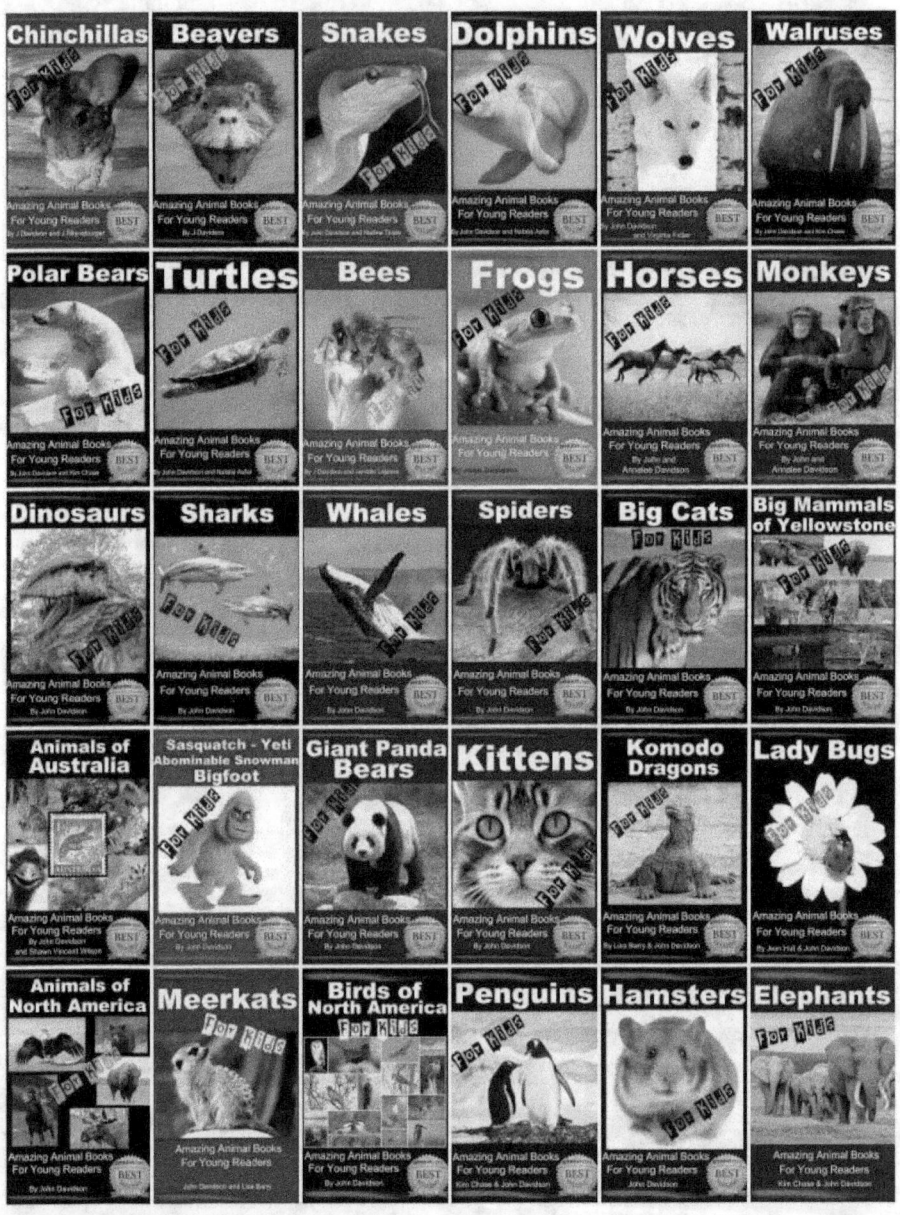

Learn To Draw Series

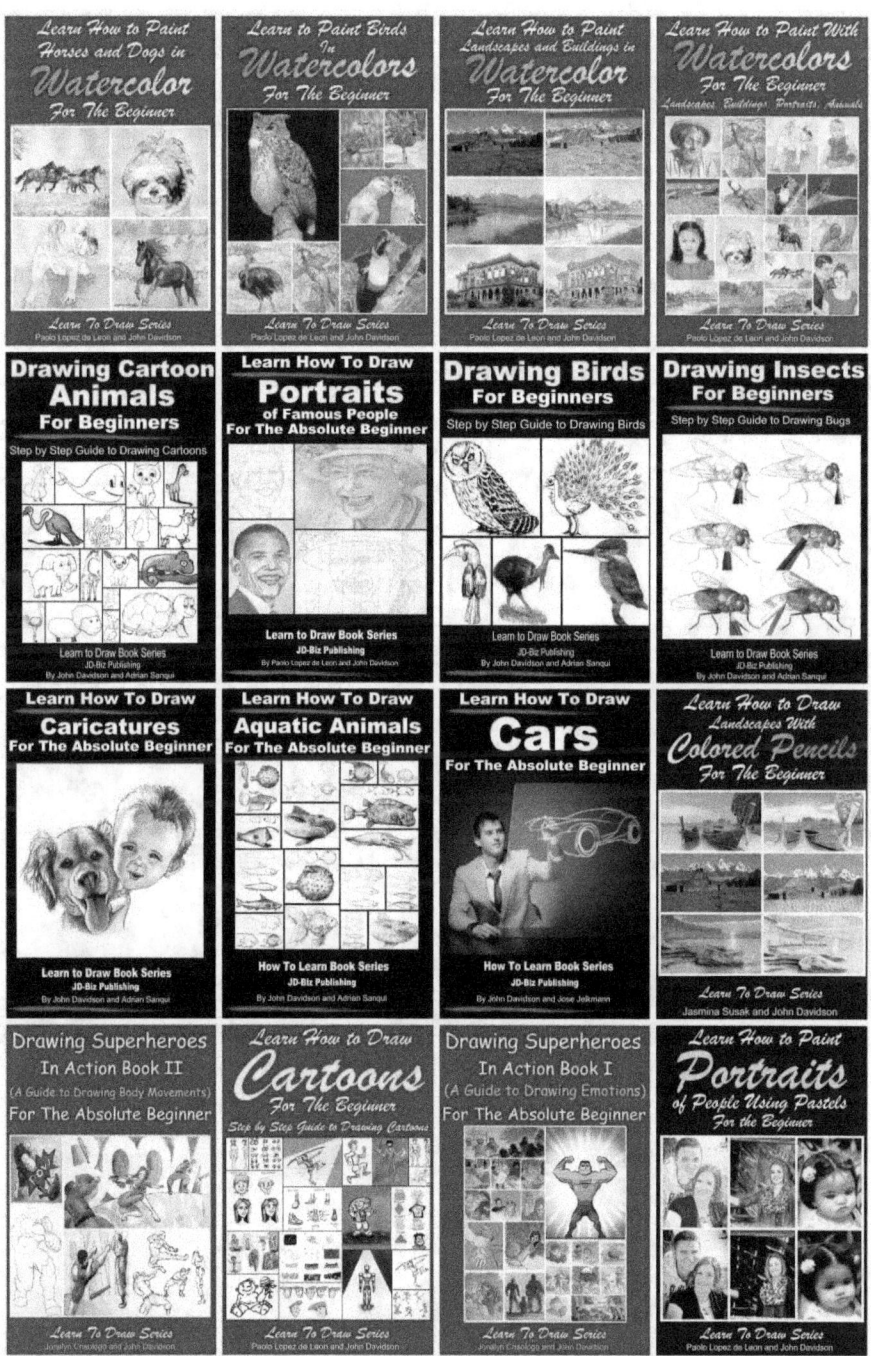

How to Build and Plan Books

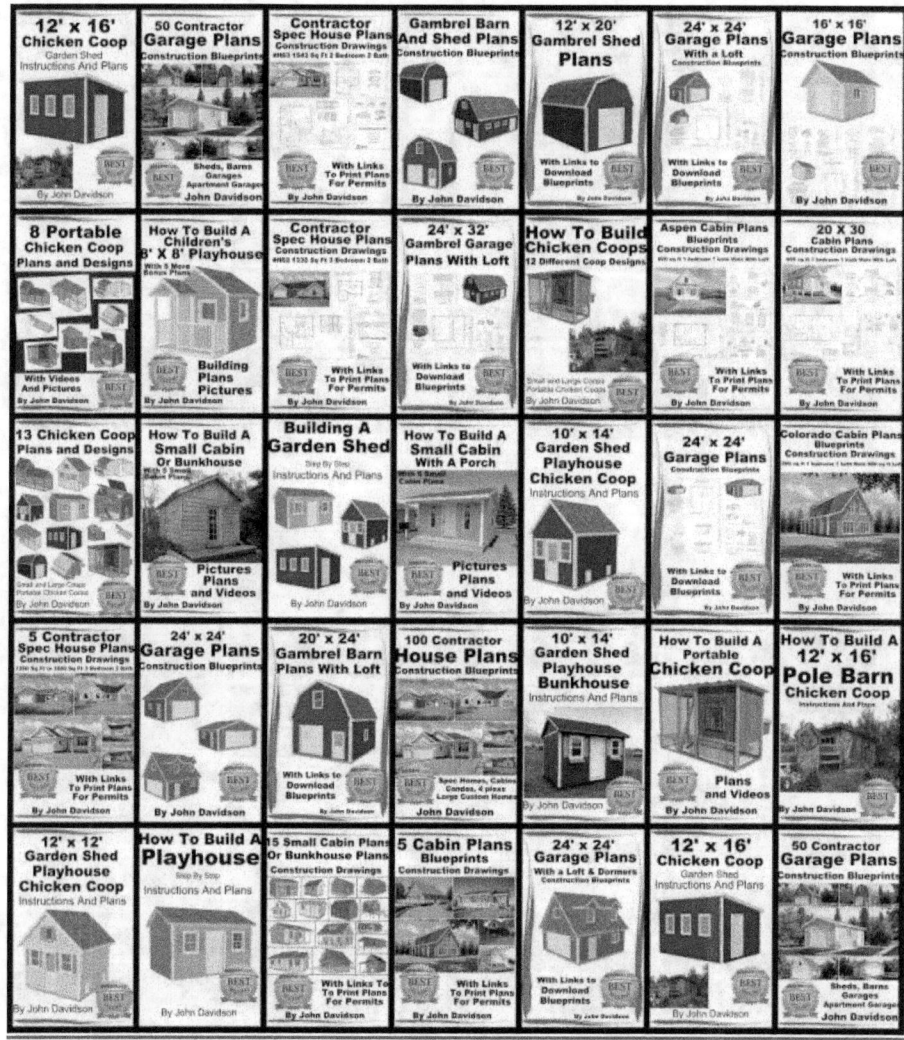

Entrepreneur Book Series

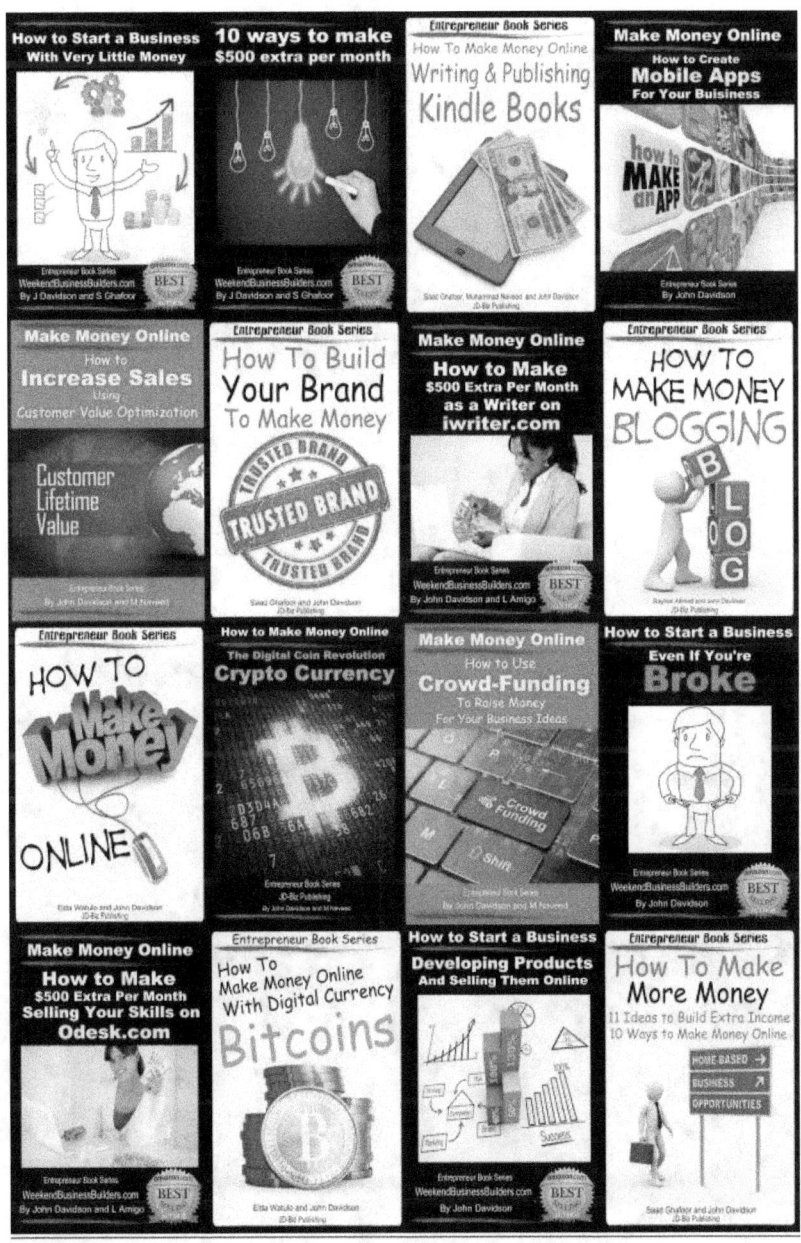

Publisher

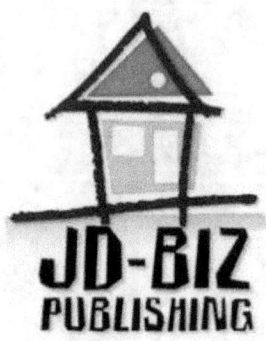

JD-Biz Corp

P O Box 374

Mendon, Utah 84325

http://www.jd-biz.com/

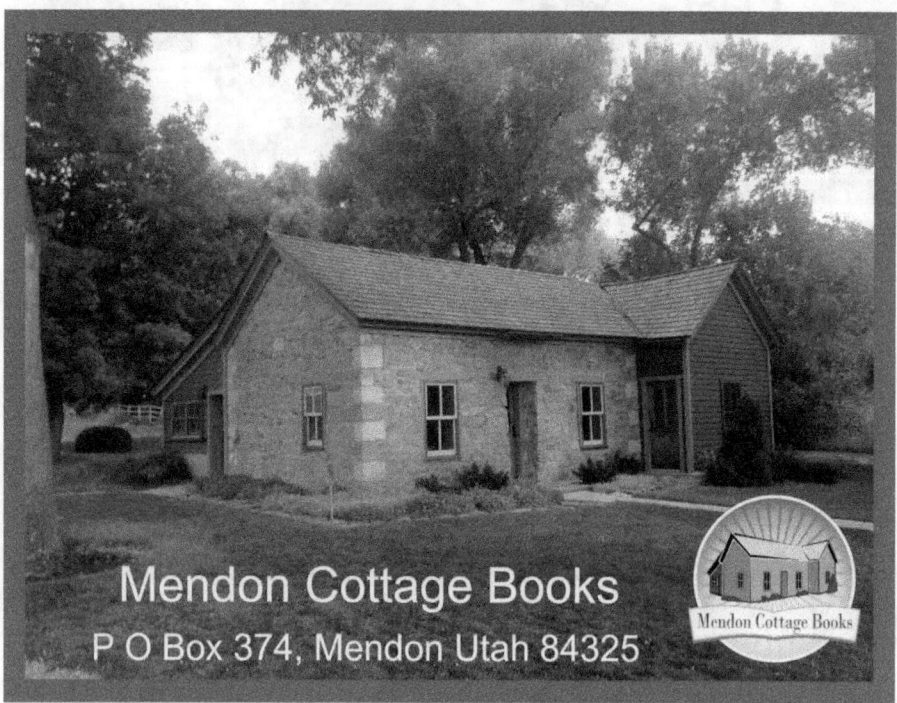

Mendon Cottage Books
P O Box 374, Mendon Utah 84325

www.ingramcontent.com/pod-product-compliance
Lightning Source LLC
Chambersburg PA
CBHW071142280526
45787CB00003B/1381

* 9 7 8 1 5 0 5 6 6 3 7 5 4 *